HEATHER FARMER

Pain in My Gut: Finding a Way Out

My journey through digestive hell and how I made it to the other side

This book was professionally typeset on Reedsy.
Find out more at reedsy.com

Contents

1

Introduction

Hi I'm Heather, and to get started, I wanted to share a little about my journey with food. Peoples' experiences with food vary widely around the world and person to person, beginning with the types of food an individual is drawn to, different foods that are available by region, and what and how much one can afford. Experiences also vary by an individual's tendency to over eat or under eat and all of the degrees and implications those partialities lead to. The last variation I'd like to get into, (one I've unfortunately had to take a very close look at because of my own experience) is the varying degrees of comfort or discomfort an individual may feel after eating.

Some people have an "iron stomach". They can eat whatever they like and enjoy every meal. I actually was in that category for much of my life, until things changed. Now, I fall into the category of one who has experienced a great deal of digestive discomfort. I know there are many out there that share my plight. There are many levels that this discomfort can take. None of them are fun, and some can slip down into very painful levels that feel brutal and torturous. Some have acid reflux which is "no picnic" of course, and down on the other end of the spectrum you have such things as ulcers and Chrones, which tend to be pretty brutal. There are many digestive issues people can have, a lot of which don't even have names, such as what I went through, and the bottom line is that they really, really suck. The low point in my journey, so far, was in 2020 when I ended up 100 lbs, (I'm 5'4" so it was pretty far down in weight) and not being able to eat or digest food at all. My digestive system had actually totally shut down for the second time in two years, so I was in continuous severe pain. This went on for a couple of days. I'm talking excruciating, level ten pain where I couldn't fall asleep or do anything else. No gas or anything else could move through my digestive system.

My first symptoms started cropping up in 2011, shortly after I tragically and traumatically lost my sister. I began waking up in the middle of the night with pain in my center upper abdomen. My doctor diagnosed it as stress and prescribed over the counter antacids. I was on and off those for years, as well as some herbal laxatives. My digestion kept getting slower and slower and more and more uncomfortable.I gradually got to a place where eating became a frightening activity because of the pain and discomfort afterwards. When my digestion shut down in 2019, I ended up in the emergency room. Between that visit and subsequent tests prescribed by a gastroenterologist, I had blood tests, a ct scan, ultrasound, and upper GI endoscopy, all of which came back clean. After all the tests, I went back to the gastroenterologist who told me, "next time take milk of magnesia." That was the brilliant diagnosis I was given. In 2020 (during the low point I just mentioned) I found myself in the emergency room again. Severe pain, digestion shut down, lots of tests, once again, no diagnosis. Not even a clue as to what was causing my symptoms.

When I looked in the mirror, I was scared. Like I said, I was 100 lbs and couldn't eat. As I peered at myself, I looked like I was skin and bones. I remember thinking "I look like someone out of a prisoner of war camp." I remember, during that time, saying to my mom,"I feel like I'm dying". It was terrifying, and I had no clue what to do. Then God, as God often does, sent me a lifeline by way of a you tube advertisement in the middle of the night. A guy who calls himself Heal Your Gut Guy. He saved my life. I bought his course, and through his program and the grace of God, crawled my way inch by inch to being able to eat again. The past four years had been a learning process of trial and error, figuring out how to actually feel good after I eat. So now I'd like to share a few of the things that have helped me, as they could possibly help someone else.

2

Confusing Advice

I've been interested in food for quite a while. My awareness of what I was putting into my body became heightened when I was around 10 years old. It was the Fourth of July gathering at my aunt and uncle's in Santa Monica, California. I was wearing a bathing suit with a hole cut in the middle, very fashionable at the time, and my big brother started teasing me about my belly getting a little bigger. I thought it was funny, but it did make me think. I also remember him teasing me when I put a lot of jelly on my toast, "that started out as a healthy piece of toast", he would kid. It was all lighthearted. He teased about a lot of little things like big brothers do. I'm very grateful now though, because it did peak my awareness. I didn't go on any diets, but I did try to eat more fruit and thought a little more in depth about the microwave pizza when I was eating it.

The thing about food these days is it can feel a little complicated. There's so much information available and so many different opinions out there. I've read about pros and cons for pretty much any food you can think of. Depending on who you talk to, meat can be the savior or the devil. Eggs are good for you one year and bad for you the next. Some say fat's good, some say it's bad. Some people don't believe in eating fruit, some want you to eat mostly fruit. The list goes on and on.

Then we can start to get into all of the different diets out there, a lot of which I've tried. In the 80's and 90's it seemed like it was all about low fat and eating pasta. I remember feeling like I was dieting and eating healthy when I would buy the fat free muffins. I also remember trying this cabbage soup diet in highschool. I felt like I was going to pass out after a couple days of doing that one.

In my early twenties I got much more into working out. It was all about protein and low carbs and trying to be as skinny as possible. After I stopped caring about being super skinny, I just ate "whatever" for many years. Somewhere in those years I did go vegan and vegetarian for a while. I did, however, arrive at the point that I was about 15 lbs overweight, so I tried a couple more diets. This was in around 2014 and 2015.

A couple of really good things stood out for me at this point though. I tried the Nutribullet diet which incorporated fresh fruits and vegetables. I started really noticing myself feeling better. My diet had gotten a little bad before that, (mostly takeout) so this was interesting to me. The other good thing was something the author in the book of another diet I was trying said. She said, "this is the year you're going to fall in love with food again", and somehow I did. I experienced some glimmers of what it would be like to love what I was eating, and found this also very interesting. Mind you, this was still a few years before my big crash, so I still had a long way to go. I do bring this up though, because I feel that the love for food is something many may have lost. I think it's something that could be rediscovered in oneself.

All that said and done, my main take away from all of this experimenting is that these days there is no easy answer to "what should I be eating?". People's body chemistry and background are different. Lifestyles are different, spiritual beliefs are different. Preferences are different. I've even heard that peoples' tastes change every 7 years. So what to do? The one piece of advice that helped me the most, came from a nutrition book I happened to read. It suggested that I needed to pay attention to how I felt after I ate. For me, that's been an important guideline. It's an important question to ask oneself in general. "How do I feel?"

3

What To Eat?

I am going to get more specific though, as to what has worked for me (some things more than "working" because some of the things I will share are what saved my life). As I've mentioned before, because of chemistry and so on, I believe it takes some trial and error to find the optimal nutrition for each individual.

So by 2019 I had managed to lose the weight I was hoping to trim off. Just a side note for anyone feeling they want to lose weight, starting a food journal was a huge factor in my success with that. I also had gotten back into yoga and working out, which was extremely helpful. The biggest problem I was having though was stress. I was going through financial problems, and overworking myself to the point of feeling totally frazzled. I believe that led me to my first emergency room visit. Then the pandemic hit and I got really sick. I struggled with respiratory illness which led to stronger and stronger antibiotics. My digestion had barely been eeking along since the previous year and ended up taking the nose dive that led to it not working at all.

The only things I'd been able to eat all of 2019 were fruit, vegetables, brown rice, and avocados. After the crash at the end of 2020 I couldn't even eat that. Even trying to drink Chamomile tea caused horrible discomfort. I was at a loss. The "Heal Your Gut Guy" course kept explaining to me that meat was actually super easy to digest. It digests quickly and early on apparently. I was skeptical and afraid. I was terrified to eat anything at that point. The thing was, that I needed to try a protein that was very easy to digest like fish. I cooked some salmon and could miraculously digest it. The other thing the course taught me was that I needed to make my grains easier to digest. I needed to break them down first. I learned to soak my brown rice in water with a splash of apple cider vinegar for 24 hours first. This breaks it down. I then cooked it with quite a bit of extra water than it calls for. I also cooked it slower and for longer than I used to so it became more like a porridge. I had to eat small bites and only a little at a time, but I was able to digest it. I was going to live.

Fruit had become very important to me over the years, and my body was longing for it. Yet again I was afraid to try anything. Something told me to cook down a banana. I put it in a pan with some water and cooked it down. I ate little bites at a time, and gradually it was ok. It tasted delicious. I think my body really needed potassium. I then learned how to make homemade applesauce, and tried a few spoons at a time. I basically had to feed my digestive system like it was a baby. Every new food I introduced had a period of adjustment, and after a while I added more and more foods from the course that my body would tolerate and accept. This was a long slow process. It took months and months before I had a decent repertoire of food I could comfortably process. In the next chapter I'll detail the basic foods I survived on and are still the foundation of my diet presently.

4

Menu Ideas

Food list and preparations:

● Protein

Chicken thighs, cook in crock pot 6 hrs with water, makes them nice and soft and easy to digest

Salmon, cook in pan or oven

Cod, oven bake is pretty easy

Halibut, easy to cook in oven (a little expensive, but so delicious once in a while)

Meatloaf (Costco and Sam's Club have bison I like to get. I use ground flax for the filler instead of breadcrumbs)

Chuck Roast, cook in crockpot with water 8-12 hrs, nice and tender

Lamb chops, (Sam's Club carries good ones for $11-12), cook in crock pot 8 hrs with water

● Grains

Brown rice, soak in water with apple cider vinegar 24 hours before cooking, extra water and cook longer (1 hr to 90 min)

Buckwheat, soak in water with apple cider vinegar 8 hours before cooking, extra water and cook longer (30-45 min)

Millet, soak in water with apple cider vinegar 24 hours before cooking, extra water and cook longer (30-45 min)

Jasmine rice, no need to soak, just rinse a few times before cooking, a little extra water and cook 20-25 min

Ezekiel bread

● Vegetables

Carrots, broccoli, cabbage, cook in pan with water until very soft Zucchini, cut into spears, cook in oven at 400 degrees for 20-30 min Beets, wrap each in foil and cook in oven at 400 degrees 1hr to 90 min Bell peppers, onions, slice and saute in pan Romaine lettuce, make into a salad

● Fruits Bananas, apples, blueberries, pears, cherries, pineapple, watermelon, grapes, lemons, limes, mangos, strawberries, dates, prunes

* Side note on fruits, in the beginning I cooked all my fruits for quite a while. I would suggest that if your digestion is in flare. Good ones to cook are: bananas, apples, blueberries, pears. Now I'm able to eat all my fruits raw.

● Dairy

Only plain greek yogurt at first, sweeten with pure maple syrup or honey When your digestion gets a little better you can try cheese once in a while and see how you do

● Nuts and seeds Chia seeds, add to plain yogurt the night before Flax seeds, grind very well Almonds, walnuts, pecans, grind in Nutribullet Macadamia nuts (very delicious)

* I was able to tolerate flax and chia pretty early on. Other nuts I didn't try until I was more healed. I suggest trying with caution.

● Homemade healthy jello (I really like the Vital Proteins Gelatin)

● Tea
   Traditional Medicinals throat coat with slippery elm, with lemon and honey. (This was all I drank for the first couple of years)
   Other teas I drink now: chamomile, roasted dandelion, ginger

What to consider limiting or avoiding: caffeine, sugar, nicotine, alcohol

These are the basic building blocks of what worked for me. I've found out through trial and error over the past four years what foods I really enjoy eating and what foods I feel really good after eating. Now they are one in the same. It's amazing to feel satisfied after each meal without any of the heaviness or discomfort. I would highly recommend checking out the Heal Your Gut Guy on you tube, as he has much more detailed information than what I've outlined here. These are just the basics of what has helped my body to heal. I don't really have full on recipes. I work full time and have to do my cooking in bulk on my days off. I then kind of mix and match throughout the week as I go. I had to eat pretty plain at first. Maybe a little butter and salt, or lemon juice and olive oil. I did gradually add in different spices and condiments, so now I have a pretty good variety of flavors. I still pretty much just cook the basics and add flavor later. My favorite is just adding some garlic or ginger to something along with salt. (Salt is important to the body, I've learned.) The best advice I could give is to be patient. And don't lose hope. I really believe the body can heal, even the digestive system.

● Spices and condiments I use now
   Garlic, ginger, italian seasoning, salad dressings (be selective and check out ingredients), mayo, mustard, soy sauce, fresh herbs (very healing), pure maple syrup (lots of good minerals), honey (also very

healing), salt

As far as what to avoid, thankfully I had given up smoking in my 20's and alcohol in 2013. I had phased out caffeine a couple of years prior by first switching to green tea, and then none all together. Sugar has been the trickiest for me the last few years. I love sweets and chocolate. At first I couldn't eat them anyways, but once I started feeling a little better, I kept adding sweets back in. Not that I felt great about it, I just kept craving them. As of the last couple weeks I've really cut back, and I do feel better. I feel I'm getting much better sleep. All these things can be really tricky to cut back on, but it's worth it if you need to heal your body. Just keep at it little by little, and you'll get to where you want to be. I learned from Louise Hay that healing the body is like cleaning a house. "You start in one room and eventually the whole house is clean."

5

Supplements

The Heal Your Gut Guy suggests several supplements in his program, but there's a couple of them that really helped get me back on my feet. The number on "go to" that I still take every day is Braggs Apple Cider Vinegar. Now I pretty much take it in the evening, but for a while I took it after most meals. You mix a tablespoon with a glass of water and drink it. It aids in digestion as well as alleviating discomfort. The other one I took religiously for a couple years was digestive enzymes. They just help your body break everything down if it's having trouble. My favorite brand is Digest Gold. I took one about 30 minutes before each meal.

A friend at work referred me to a really good chiropractor during this time. He was kind of a naturopath of sorts and was very helpful. He recommended I take marshmallow root each evening to help rebuild the lining in my stomach and intestines. I stuck with that for a couple of months and it really helped.

Probiotics were the next biggie. The program I learned from didn't recommend them right away because I was in such a bad flare up. Once things calmed down a bit I started on some excellent ones that made a huge difference for me. Probiotics help rebuild the microbiome in your gut. This in turn helps your immune system, your digestion, as well as your emotions. The most imperative thing I needed help with was my regularity. I was in a never ending state of fear of becoming constipated. It was awful. Once I was able to get on a good regimen of probiotics, that worry finally went away. There is one I get on Amazon that is wonderful called Just Thrive. There is also a company called Amare. I order their FundaMentals Pack and take that on a regular basis. I alternate between the two, but what a world of difference they made to me.

I had also heard that magnesium helps with constipation. I definitely needed all the help I could get. I somehow stumbled on liquid magnesium, and it was such a life saver. I still take it every night. Magnesium is also good for muscles and has a calming effect, it's a great nightly regimen. The main thing is that it's extremely helpful with regularity. I love the Trace Minerals liquid magnesium. I take three dropfuls every evening with water, and highly recommend it.

Lastly, I regularly take a nice multivitamin. That's just a practice I've kept up for many, many years now. Just to cover my bases, so to speak. Amare has a great multivitamin, and it's in capsule form, which my niece tells me is the most efficient form, since it breaks down easier.

6

Helpful Tips

Finding my way back to a place where I could comfortably digest food has been like finding pieces of a puzzle and gradually putting them together. What types of food to eat, how to prepare them, and what supplements to take are some very important pieces, but there are more. There is one really important one that can be very difficult to figure out. It may even be the most difficult, but I believe it to be hugely important.

Portion size. It's a tricky one. We just believe we need to eat more than we actually do. It's instilled in our culture as well as our instincts. I learned from the "HYGG" course that the prophet Muhammed taught long ago to fill the stomach only one third full with food. This will leave one third left for a drink and one third for air. This will lead to optimal digestion.This equals around one to two cups of food in one sitting. Culturally speaking, start noticing the amount of food you receive at a restaurant. Many times it's much more than that. The trick I'm trying to work with myself on is eating half and taking the other half home. It's not easy to do. If something tastes good, I just want to keep eating. This isn't a fault either. It's a brilliant survival instinct that came from my predecessors roaming in the wild, and not knowing where their next meal was coming from. The only thing I can do is practice with my portion sizes until I get it down, because when I have a day where I've eaten the right portion sizes all day, I feel a million times better. Especially when I've eaten healthy foods and gotten great nutrition for the day!

The next puzzle piece is something I'm finally getting into a good habit of doing. It is also pretty tricky because most of what we are used to when it comes to a typical meal goes against it. This philosophy comes from an older book that I read a long time ago, but the principles always stuck in the back of my head for some reason. The book it's called "Living Health", by Harvey and Marilyn Diamond. They recommend certain food combinations. Basically you don't eat protein and starch in the same meal. The science behind it is that the chemistry to digest each one is different, basically making digestion much more difficult when eaten together. It took a lot of practice, but I've finally been able to implement this pretty regularly. It does feel amazing, actually. Most days (I try not to be extremely rigid with anything) I eat just a protein and vegetable for lunch, and a starch and vegetable for dinner. I eat fruit first thing in the morning (another principle they recommend). I have a few things I like for breakfast, usually yogurt, Ezekiel bread, or smoothies. One of the best things about food combining is how much easier it makes portion size. The best thing though, is how much better you will feel after you eat. It's so worth giving it a try. Please do!

The last little bit of fine tuning I've been working on lately comes from another book that I read years back, and recently became interested in. It's called "Eat Right For Your Type" by Dr. Peter J D'Adamo. The basic philosophy is that, depending on your blood type, different foods will react with your body's chemistry more positively or negatively than other foods. I highly recommend checking out the book for your type, just to experiment if anything. I don't stick to it as a hard and fast rule, as the book doesn't even suggest doing that. I have been trending towards more of the foods that are supposed to work well with my type. I think that the improvements I've felt by following this book are a little more subtle, but I have noticed an overall increase in my energy levels.

7

Other Factors

So far, we've talked about what to eat and what to put in the body. These things are so important to me and they saved my life. There are other influences though, that can profoundly affect your digestive system. One of them being movement. This can be extremely challenging for someone who isn't feeling well, but I can't stress enough how important it is to find a way to move. I found a yoga practice I was able to do. It's called Yoga For Health with Jenny Cornero: Gastro-Intestinal Disorders. It was free on my local library streaming service. The first year or so after my digestive collapse, I had to go through a lot of trial and error figuring out what and how to eat. I still experienced discomfort much of the time. Every time I introduced any new food it was rough at first. I was just trying to make it through the day most days and it wasn't easy. In fact it was hard as hell. This yoga practice got me over the humps. I managed to do it a couple of times a week, and it pulled me through.

Yoga poses basically massage the digestive organs. This increases the circulation, helping to heal the organs as well as helping to move the food through the digestive tract. The other helpful thing about yoga is the effect it has on the nervous system. When the body is stressed, the part of the nervous system called SNS is active. That is your "flight or fight" response. When this system is going wild, your digestion decreases. The PNS part of the system is taking over more when you are relaxed. This is the one getting your digestion working well. It's commonly referred to as "rest and digest". According to an article in PubMed Central "yoga's beneficial effect in accentuating the PNS over the SNS has long been known". Even if you just start with 5 min of yoga and work your way up, it could be a game changer. It was for me.

The shape I was in those first few months was pretty feeble. When I went back to work my legs could barely get me from my car to the building, they were so shaky and weak. Climbing a flight of stairs felt like climbing a mountain. I kept pushing through and gradually they regained strength. However, exercise just wasn't doable for me those first few months. I knew I would make it back to exercising though. I consider myself very fortunate because I grew up with grandparents and parents who exercised. When I was in high school my big brother used to take me and my brother to the gym with him. My first job was at a gym and no matter how difunctional my life has ever been, I always come back to exercise at some point. It's a saving grace and I'm so thankful for it.

Whenever and however you can do it, try to get some physical activity into your life. Moving around improves your digestion. The list of the benefits of exercise goes on and on: it stimulates gastric motility, boosts the number of healthy gut bacteria, reduces the risk of colon cancer, improves quality of life in those with IBS, relieves constipation, prevents gallstones,and improves your gut microbiome composition, just to name a few. The other thing you will improve is your emotions, which in turn will have a positive effect on your digestion. With exercise you will increase the proficiency of your neurotransmitters. This is your serotonin, dopamine, norepinephrine, and endorphins etc. This will reduce your anxiety, depression, and stress. It will increase your feelings of well being and relaxation. This will help your PNS, which will, as we said before, help to heal your digestion. I found streaming short workouts at home was the easiest way for me to start adding exercise back into my life. I started off slow with what little I could do and built it up.

8

Stress Relief

I'd like to continue a little further into emotions and relaxation. The bottom line is that we live in a very stressful world. For most people the stress never stops. Stress on its own isn't actually a negative thing. In fact we need it and that's part of how we grow. The problem comes from stress overload,when it just goes on and on, and there's little if any relief. My belief is that this is a major factor in disease. I strongly believe in the body's natural ability to heal itself, not only because of everything I've read, but also because of the amount of things in my own body that I've witnessed healing. We just have to give our body the chance. I love life and I love to do a lot of things, but sometimes we need to slow down. I think of our stressful busy lives as "go, go, go" and sometimes we just need to take it back the other way.

I have a few suggestions on how we can do that.

● Massages

I am a massage therapist by trade and I definitely take my own advice. Getting a massage is one of the best ways to stimulate your PNS. This lowers your heart rate, blood pressure, and stress levels, and promotes relaxation and healing. I do get a massage once a month myself, but even a couple times a year can have great benefits.

● Meditation

Meditation is such a great stress reliever. It's much easier and more doable than you would think. Just find a quiet place to lie down. Get comfy, put your headphones on and find a meditation on you tube to listen to. I've been doing this for years and it can be a lifesaver if you're having trouble sleeping.

● Steam room, sauna, jacuzzis

If you have any spas or gyms in your area with these amenities, it can be such a relaxing activity. Just sit, unwind, and let your stress melt away.

● Nature

Just getting any time outside has a very relaxing effect. Whether going to the park or just sitting in your yard, it helps a lot just to get some air from time to time.

● Limiting screen time

I know this one can be super challenging but I think it really helps to take a break here and there. If only just in the evenings for a bit right before bed. The eyes just need that rest. I suggest switching to listening to an audiobook about a half an hour or more before bed.

● Sleep

Getting enough sleep is a big deal for your digestion. The amount of sleep required varies by individual, so the exact time will vary. I've just noticed that when I don't get enough, my digestion definitely doesn't work as well.

9

Conclusion

Where am I now? Well, my digestion isn't perfect. I'm definitely still a work in progress. Most days it's pretty good though, and some days it's excellent. So, I will continue on. Thank you for going on my journey with me.

I know digestive troubles can be hellish and awful. I know there is hope though. Please don't give up. My best advice is something I've learned from going through horrible, difficult times, and that is take care of yourself. Find any tiny thing that gives you even the smallest amount of comfort. Whether it's a tv show, heating pad, comfy pajamas, or a bath. Just find something that makes things a little better and give that to yourself. Find a way to give yourself a little love. You only need to make it through each day, one day at a time, and you can do it!

If you found this book to be helpful, I'd be very appreciative if you left a favorable review on Amazon!

10

References

Guy, H. Y. G. (n.d.). FULL 4-STEP Mike Method - Heal your gut guy. https://healyourgutguy.com/

National Center for Biotechnology Information. (n.d.). https://ncbi.nlm.nih.gov/

Top gastroenterologist in Plano TX | Arshad Malik, MD. (n.d.). https://arshadmalikmd.com/

Diamond, H., & Diamond, M. (1989).

Living health. D'Adamo, P. J., & Whitney, C. (2016). Eat right 4 Your type (Revised and updated): The Individualized Blood Type Diet® Solution. Penguin